50 WAYS *TO* TREAT KIDNEY STONES

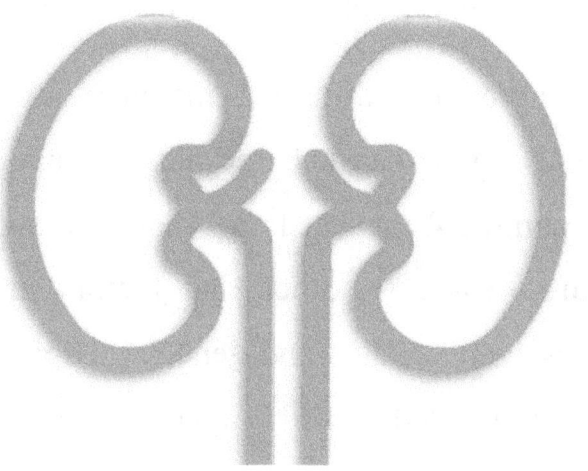

BY AMELIA AVA

INTRODUCTION

Around 10% of the world's population is affected by kidney disease, a prevalent condition. The kidneys are powerful, small, bean-shaped organs that carry out numerous essential functions. They are in charge of a lot of important things, like filtering out waste, releasing hormones that control blood pressure, keeping the body's fluids in balance, and making urine.

There are different manners by which these essential organs can become harmed. Kidney disease is most commonly caused by diabetes and high blood pressure. However, other risk factors include obesity, smoking, gender, age, and genetics. High blood pressure and uncontrolled blood sugar damage kidney blood vessels, reducing their capacity for optimal function.

Waste, including food waste, accumulates in the blood when the kidneys are not functioning properly. Your kidneys separate waste and excess fluid from your blood so that they can be excreted in your urine. Kidney failure occurs when your kidneys stop working and are unable to perform their functions.

The revolutionary treatment that you are about to learn about on this page is twice as effective as the most popular drugs for kidney problems in getting rid of infections, getting rid of kidney stones, and alleviating back pain.

Thousands of people around the world have successfully implemented this strategy, which has assisted them in treating their kidney condition and restoring their health. If you are a man or woman in your forties, fifties, sixties, or seventies, there is a very good chance that you will be experiencing a variety of common symptoms, including the following:

- ❖ Sharp Pain: You keep getting this sharp pain that comes and goes in your back, belly, and waist side. The pain changes where it is and how bad it is.
- ❖ Desperation - You just barely went to the latrine 30 minutes prior yet you want to pee once more.

- ❖ You feel like a detainee in your own home, unfit to move more than 100ft from the closest toilet
- ❖ Swelling: Your legs, feet, and ankles are swelling, along with a puffy face, nausea, and vomiting.
- ❖ Urinary Burning: When you urinate, you just feel this burning pain.
- ❖ Bloody Urine: You just used the bathroom, and you notice that your urine is brown, pink, and red. Additionally, you notice that it is cloudy, foamy, and odorous.
- ❖ Weak Flow: Eventually, you find release and begin a flow; however, it is barely moving, it drips, it stops and starts, and it is simply not what it should be.

Infection and kidney stones are not only painful, but they can also be embarrassing. To exacerbate the situation, the condition can prompt hazardous confusions.

Kidney Stones can prompt further confusion in future on the off chance that you don't treat it now. By clogging your kidneys with urine, it causes blockage. Acute urinary retention may occur in these situations.

It may even progress to chronic kidney disease, kidney damage or infection, damage to the bladder, and stones in the bladder.

THE BASICS

In this first set of advice, some of the fundamentals of kidney stones will be discussed.

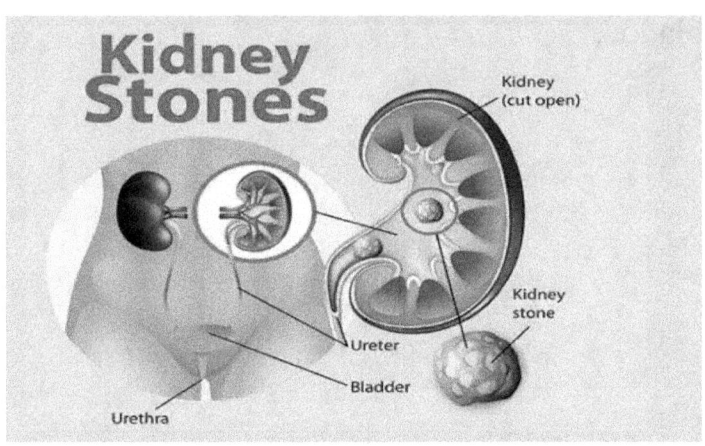

1. Definition

The formation of crystals on the kidneys by minerals and other substances in excessively concentrated urine is what causes kidney stones.

Stones or small, hard masses can result from the combination of these crystals. The majority of kidney stones do not cause any damage to your bladder over time; however, some cause severe pain and necessitate surgery.

2. History

Kidney stones date back to the time of the Egyptian pyramids and continue to be a prevalent condition today. In fact, the number of kidney stones has increased steadily over time.

3. Symptoms

Kidney stones can occur without causing symptoms. If you do notice anything, it probably indicates a blockage. Some of the more typical symptoms include:

- ❖ A sharp pain that can last anywhere from five to fifteen minutes.
- ❖ Urine that is cloudy, bloody, or sour-tasting
- ❖ Vomiting and nausea
- ❖ Persistent urge to urinate
- ❖ Chills and fever

4. Causes

Kidney stones can be caused by a variety of factors, including:

- ❖ Genetics
- ❖ Factors affecting one's lifestyle
- ❖ Medical conditions
- ❖ Diet
- ❖ Drugs
- ❖ Climate Anticipation

5. Preventions

There are loads of things that you can do that will forestall your gamble of getting kidney stones

A lot of these only require a few adjustments to one's way of life. Later on in this eBook, we'll talk more about these changes in lifestyle.

TYPES

In the following set of advice, we'll talk about the four different kinds of kidney stones.

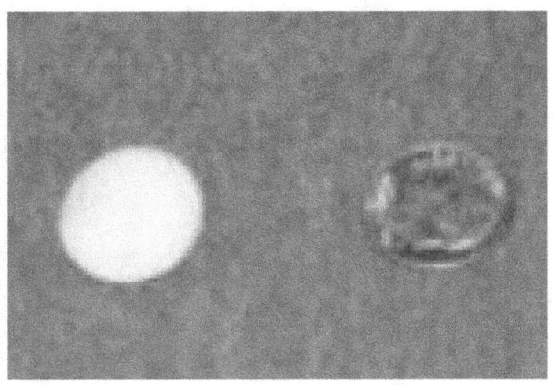

6. Calcium Stones:

Calcium stones account for about four out of every five kidney stones.

Most of these stones are made of calcium and oxalate mixed together. Oxalate is found naturally in some vegetables and fruits.

7. Struvite Stones

Consistent infections of the urinary tract are almost always the cause of struvite stones. Women are more likely than men to have struvite stones. They develop into struvite stones as a result of an elevated level of ammonia in the urine.

They can seriously harm your kidneys and tend to be large and horn-shaped.

8. Uric Corrosive Stones

These stones are shaped of uric corrosive, a result of protein digestion. If you have had chemotherapy, consume a high-protein diet, or have certain genetic factors that predispose you to the condition, you are more likely to develop uric acid stones.

9. Cystine Stones

Cystine stones affect very few people. Typically, they are brought on by a genetic condition. Cystinuria is a condition in which the kidneys secrete a lot of certain amino acids.

RISK FACTORS

The following set of advice will go over the risk factors for kidney stones.

Kidney stones are more likely to occur in people who have a history of kidney stones. You are more likely to develop kidney stones if a family member does. Additionally, if you have kidney stones in the past, you may develop them again.

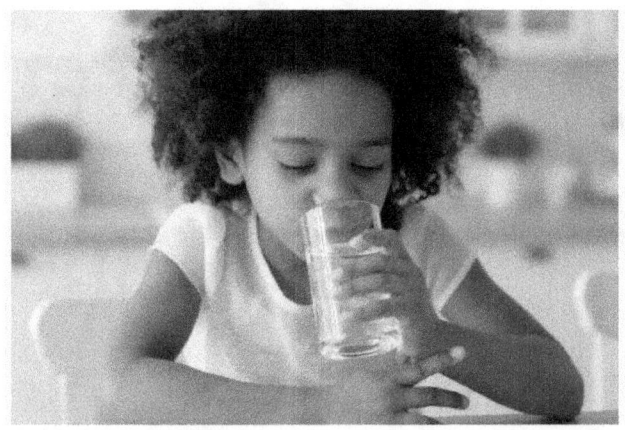

10. Insufficient Fluids:

If you don't drink enough fluids, you run the risk of developing kidney stones. Additionally, working or living in a hot, dry environment increases your risk because you lose fluids more quickly.

11. Diet

Your diet may increase your risk of kidney stones.

For instance, eating a lot of sodium (salt) and protein (meat, chicken, and fish) increases your risk of developing kidney stones.

12. Age, Race, and Sex

The following data about kidney stones are grouped by sex, race, and age:

- Between the ages of 20 and 70, kidney stones affect the majority of people.
- Kidney stones are more common in men than in women.
- White Americans are more likely than black Americans to develop kidney stones.

13. Drugs

Some drugs can make you more likely to get kidney stones.

In some cases, diuretics, for instance, can make you more likely to get kidney stones. Make sure to discuss all of your medications with your doctor.

14. Diseases

You may be more likely to develop kidney stones if you have rare conditions like cystinuria and renal tubular acidosis. Kidney stones can also be caused by more common conditions like hyperparathyroidism, chronic urinary tract infections, and gout.

15. Activity

A lack of physical activity can cause your bones to release more calcium, increasing your risk of kidney stones. If you're out of commission or extremely fixed for an extensive stretch of time, you're at a greater gamble.

DIAGNOSING

In the following set of advice, we'll talk about how kidney stones are found.

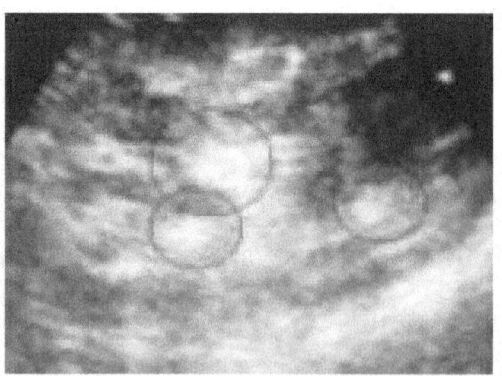

16. X-ray

Your doctor may order an X-ray if he thinks you have kidney stones. Most kidney stones can be seen on an abdominal X-ray, which can also help the doctor determine how the size of the stone has changed over time.

17. Ultrasound

Instead of X-rays, some doctors use ultrasounds. An ultrasound is noninvasive, safe, and without pain. It may miss smaller stones, which is a drawback.

18. Intravenous Pyelography

In an intravenous pyelography, contrast dye is injected into an arm vein. As the dye moves through your kidneys, ureters, and bladder, a series of X-rays are taken.

19. CT Scan

The evaluation of kidney stones using a CT scan has pretty much become the norm. It is a quick test that does not require contrast dye and can identify even the tiniest stones. The downside is that it costs a lot.

TREATMENT

This next set of tips will talk about some of the treatment choices accessible for individuals with kidney stones.

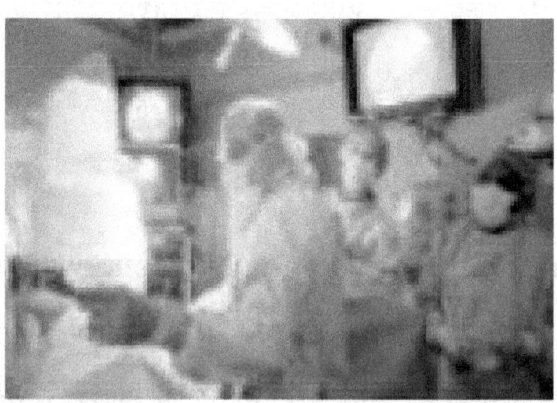

20. Extracorporeal Shock Wave Lithotripsy (ESWL)

The procedure known as extracorporeal shock wave lithotripsy (ESWL) is frequently utilized for the treatment of kidney stones. It breaks the stones up into small pieces with shock waves, which are then excreted in your urine. Sedation or light anesthesia are typically required for ESWL patients.

21. Percutaneous Nephrolithotomy

If ESWL is unsuccessful, your surgeon may need to use a nephroscope to remove your kidney stone through a small incision in your back. The procedure is known as a Percutaneous Nephrolithotomy.

22. Ureterscopic Stone Removal

To remove a stone that has become lodged in the ureter, a ureterscopic stone removal procedure is carried out. An ureteroscope, a small instrument, is used to catch the stone during this procedure.

A ultrasound can likewise be put through the degree to break the stone.

23. Overactive Parathyroid Glands

Overactive parathyroid glands, which are a part of your thyroid gland, can lead to some calcium stones. Parathyroid surgery Kidney stones are the result of this excess calcium. The issue can be resolved through parathyroid surgery.

24. Neuropathic Treatment

Nutrition is the primary focus of neuropathic treatment. A lot of people think that eating well can help the kidneys work well and prevent stones from forming.

MEDICATIONS

For each of the four types of kidney stones, distinct medications are available. The medications that are used to treat each type will be listed in the following set of advice.

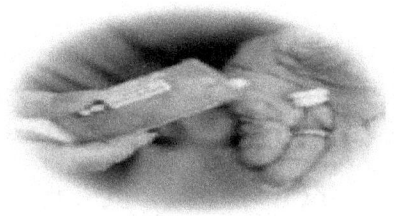

25. Calcium Stones

Thiazide diuretics may be prescribed by your doctor if you are prone to calcium stones. Your doctor may prescribe sodium or potassium bicarbonate if renal tubular acidosis is the cause of your calcium stones.

26. Struvite Stones

Antibiotics are used to treat and prevent struvite stones because they are caused by bacteria in the urine. To prevent kidney stones in the future, your doctor may recommend taking antibiotics in small doses for a long time.

27. Uric Acid Stones

Your doctor may prescribe Zyloprim or Aloprim to treat uric acid stones. Your blood and urine levels of uric acid are reduced by these medications.

28. Cystine Stones

Because they are the hardest, cystine stones are the most challenging to treat. In addition to recommending an extremely high urine output, your doctor may recommend medications to alkalize the urine.

THINGS YOU CAN DO AT HOME

There are a number of things you can do at home to treat kidney stones and even prevent them. This next set of tips will examine a portion of these.

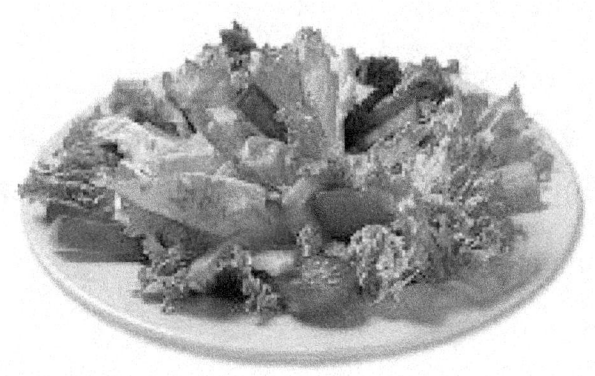

29. Drinking water

Drinking water is probably one of the simplest things you can do to reduce your risk of developing kidney stones. Every day, you should consume at least half of your body weight in ounces of water. For instance, a 150 lb individual would hydrate.

30. Eat well

Eat well Consuming healthy foods can lower your risk of kidney stones. Things like:

- Green leafy vegetables,
- Fruits, whole grains
- Legumes, small amounts of fish and poultry
- Brown rice
- Bananas
- Oats,
- Barley

31. Stay Active

Regular exercise can aid in the prevention of kidney stones. Studies have shown that individuals who lead dynamic

ways of life are more averse to foster kidney stones. To lower your risk, get active on a daily basis.

32. Pack of Castor Oil

Pack of Castor Oil Castor oil can be used to alleviate painful cramping or spasms because it has anti-inflammatory properties. Put a towel that has been soaked in castor oil where it hurts

33. Hot Pack

To make a pack, hot Pack the tense muscles caused by kidney stone pain can be relaxed with a hot pack. They can also make it easier for the stones to pass.

34. Hot Vinegar

Additionally, hot vinegar can alleviate the severe pain caused by kidney stones. Place a towel over the painful area that has been soaked in a 50:50 vinegar: water solution.

35. Limiting Oxalates

Limiting Oxalates Limiting oxalates-rich foods can help prevent kidney stones. Some of these foods are:

- ❖ Okra
- ❖ Beets

- Collards
- Refried beans
- Spinach
- Sweet potatoes

36. Cautious about L-ascorbic Acid

A few investigations show that really limiting your L-ascorbic acid utilization, it might assist with forestalling kidney stones. Oxalate production can rise if consumed in excess of 3 to 4 grams per day, increasing the risk of kidney stones.

37. Watch out for vitamin D

Watch out for vitamin D Excess vitamin D can increase the risk of kidney stones. Calcium can be too much from vitamin D, putting you at risk for kidney stones. Vitamin D intake should never exceed 400 IU per day.

38. Other Things to Avoid

Other Things to Avoid Additional things to avoid to reduce your risk of developing kidney stones are:

Sugar, antacids, too much protein, dairy products, salt, carbonated drinks, caffeine.

39. Myth About Oral Calcium

Reducing your calcium intake does not appear to lower your risk. Women who consume more calcium have a lower risk of developing kidney stones than women who consume less calcium, according to research. Roper

HERBAL REMEDIES AND SUPPLEMENTS

In the final set of advice, we'll talk about some herbal remedies and supplements for kidney stones.

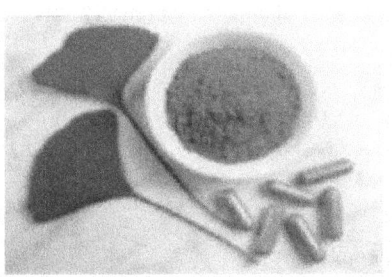

40. Magnesium Citrate

A lack of magnesium intake has been linked to a high risk of kidney stones, according to research. Supplementing with magnesium may not only reduce the size of existing stones but also prevent new ones from *forming.500 mg per day is a good dose.

41. Vitamin B-6

A deficiency in vitamin B-6 has been linked to an increa/se in urinary oxalate, which may result in kidney stones.25 mg per day is a good dose.

42. Vitamin

A has been shown to treat and prevent kidney stones in foods high in vitamin A. Some examples of these foods are:

43. Bearberry

The evergreen shrub bearberry can be used as a urinary tract diuretic and antiseptic. It has long been used to treat bladder or urinary tract infections. Bearberry can be purchased in capsules or as a tea in a health food store.

44. Cleavers

Cleavers have a long history of treating urinary infections, stones, and congestive kidney disorders. Clivers, Goosegrass, and Bedstraw are all other names for cleavers. They are available at any herbal store.

45. Corn Silk

Corn silk is utilized to alleviate kidney stone pain. Additionally, it has a mild diuretic effect. Corn-silk can be purchased at your neighborhood herbal store to heal your kidneys and increase urine flow.

46. Cramp Bark

Cramp Bark is an antispasmodic and used to relax smooth muscles. Kidney stone pain is significantly reduced by this. Again, you can get this from a health food or herbal store.

47. Gravel Root

Numerous conditions, including kidney stones, can be treated with gravel root. Additionally, it aids in the following conditions:

- ❖ Urinary diseases
- ❖ Prostatitis
- ❖ Pelvic fiery infection
- ❖ Ailment
- ❖ Gout

48. Khella

Khella has been treating kidney stones for quite a while.

According to research, the khella relaxes the ureter tissue, making it easier for smaller stones to pass.

49. Seven Barks

Seven Barks is a herb that relaxes the urinary system. Seven barks are a plant. It relaxes the body, making it easier to get rid of kidney stones.

50. Stone Root

Stone root is a potent diuretic that has a history of both assisting in the removal of kidney stones and preventing the formation of new ones.

www.ingramcontent.com/pod-product-compliance
Lightning Source LLC
Chambersburg PA
CBHW050327220526
45465CB00005B/2161